The CHRISTIAN FAMILY CAREGIVER

DEVOTIONAL

The
CHRISTIAN FAMILY CAREGIVER
DEVOTIONAL

FINDING JOY IN THE JOURNEY AS
YOU CARE FOR YOUR LOVED ONE

Evelyn Olsen, RN CMC

Contents

This book is a love offering to Aunt Pat, whose kind, radiant, indomitable spirit continues to inspire all of us who know her. Thank you for trusting me to be your caregiver and confidant. For the last two decades, you've been my number one fan, urging me with your trademark phrase, 'You have to write a book.' Well, Aunt Pat, here it is...the first one, and I'm dedicating it to you!

Introduction

Taking on the role of family caregiver for an aging loved one is a commendable and compassionate decision. However, this path is not without its significant challenges and obstacles. This book is crafted in a daily devotional style chock full of valuable insights for family caregivers. Yet even though it is in the style of a daily devotional, I'd like to extend a warm invitation to you to read it at your own pace. Rushing through the content is discouraged. Take your time, savor each day, and allow the wisdom within to seep into your consciousness.

As a fellow family caregiver, I understand the time constraints and the constant demands on your schedule. It's tough to set aside dedicated time for personal reflection and growth, so there's no need to cram yourself into a rigid schedule to finish this book quickly. We all have enough on our plates already.

Instead, let this book be your companion, one that you can return to at your own convenience. The truth is that on some days, you'll manage to set aside time for reading and contemplation, while on others, your schedule may be too hectic to allow that much-needed personal time. Like many of us, I've experienced days when even a moment in the bathroom felt like a rare luxury.

As family caregivers, we need to support each other; therefore, it's essential that we stick together; otherwise, we might fall apart. We're all in the same boat, and we know what it's like to walk in our own boat shoes. Even when others can't fathom the journey we're on, we get it, and we talk the same lingo. We're the ones the crew depends on to keep the ship afloat even while navigating rough waters and tumultuous winds.

If it takes more than 30 days to get through these pages, that's perfectly fine. Go at your own pace, and don't rush. This means finding some space whenever you can to do what ya gotta do. Just do your best while walking out the calling of caring for your loved one. Be sure, however, not to forget the importance of tending to yourself. If you leave yourself simmering on the back burner, too, without an occasional stir, you'll get overdone, become scorched, and ultimately burn out. Burnout, also called Care Fatigue or Compassion Fatigue, is real, and it's no fun...for anyone. I can personally attest to that, having been hospitalized twice for Adrenal Exhaustion. Always remember the airplane safety analogy—put your oxygen mask on first before assisting others. It's vital for your well-being and your ability to provide care. Your goal should be to absorb the wisdom and insights in this book and not to complete the book in record time. Your preferred style of reading and comprehension is what matters most.

My prayer for you as you read and contemplate is that God will grant you the wisdom, knowledge, and understanding you need to be the healthiest family caregiver and person you can be and that your life will glorify Him. I pray that God will inevitably make a way where there seems to be no way when you can't find time to rest and that you will know that the time of the day is not as important as just making time whenever you can.

No guilt. You Do you. Remember, your journey through this book is a personal one, and I hope it enriches your life and your caregiving journey as well.

Day 1: Love as Your Compass

NAVIGATING THE CAREGIVING JOURNEY

"Above all, love each other deeply because love covers a multitude of sins." - 1 Peter 4:8

Hello to you fellow caregivers, and welcome to Day One of our incredible journey. Today, we're setting our compass to love, the True North in the World of Caring.

Let's travel this journey together and think of it as a thrilling, learning adventure where love is both the map and the destination.

> "Love is not something you merely feel;
> it's something you do."
> - David Wilkerson

Personal Reflections:

In all my years as a caregiver, I've learned to rely on Love as my unwavering compass. It's been my constant companion on this caregiving journey. Whenever I find myself navigating the twists and turns of this rugged path, I don't lose my cool. No, siree! I simply pull out my Love Compass and seek my True North. It's like a GPS, always pointing upwards towards clarity and the right direction. So, fellow travelers, even in the wildest caregiving terrains, remember that your Love Compass forever guides you towards the North – embrace it, and you'll always find your way to your destiny!

Today, let's embrace this journey with open hearts, ready to pour out love in every task, every smile, and every act of care.

The Word of God tells us that when we truly love someone, we will overlook their faults and mistakes. This brings to my mind a story involving Noah's 3 sons. Even though all three were of the same family, they were unlike. While Ham showed disrespect towards his father by gazing at his nakedness, Shem and Japheth demonstrated profound love and compassion by looking away and covering him up when he was lying inebriated and naked. The action of Shem and Japheth was a powerful symbol of love's ability to protect, forgive, unify, and restore. Their protective gesture conveyed care and benevolent love, offering redemption and solidarity even in the moment of their father Noah's vulnerability and sin. This biblical tale is one example of many that underscore Christian virtues, emphasizing forgiveness, grace, and the significance of extending compassion and understanding to others, which reflects a Christ-like love that transcends judgment.

Sensing the love of others is a fundamental human need. This is why each person needs to be seen, validated, and embraced by the people they hold dear. These needs are as essential to us as our requirements for nourishment and hydration

The primary objective of understanding your loved ones' love languages is to cultivate selflessness. Becoming more selfless rather than selfish is what Jesus meant when he said, "Whoever wants to be my disciple deny themselves and take up their cross and follow me." It's about shifting the focus from our own preferences to theirs by deliberately seeking to communicate love in the way that resonates most deeply with them. In doing so, we foster a deeper connection, empathy, and a selfless, nurturing bond that nourishes both the giver and the receiver of love.

Each person has their own distinct love language, and it's crucial to delve into and comprehend these languages. This discovery not only strengthens our bonds but also fosters a deeper connection. In the realm of caregiving, where trust is paramount, this connection becomes an invaluable asset. Remember, countless ways exist to express love and care for those we cherish.

Love languages are not rigid, and people may have different preferences. There is actually an official Love Language quiz that can provide us with a clear answer; however, there are many other ways to uncover what can make our loved one purr without knowing the results of a quiz.

Discovering our loved one's Love Language is like uncovering a precious gem in a treasure hunt. It will have you saying, "Ah hah…I found what makes them tick!"

Practical Applications:

1. Read the following list and learn what the **5 Love Languages** are.
2. Once you've learned what they are, delve deeper to determine which one or ones might be applicable to your loved one's situation.
3. Take into account which of the following appears to align most closely with your loved one's behaviors.

Following is the list of the 5 Love Languages, accompanied by some suggestions to assist you in identifying which ones might be relevant to your loved one's preferences:

GIFTS:

Gifts in Kind: Instead of Cash, you might have noticed that your loved one frequently gives thoughtful presents or treasures to others. This may indicate that they appreciate the love language of giving and receiving gifts.

Expressive Giving: Pay attention to how they express affection through gifts. If they have a knack for finding meaningful gifts and celebrating special occasions with presents, it's a telltale sign.

Thoughtful Tokens: Look for their importance on the thought behind the gift rather than the value. If your loved one values the sentiment and thoughtfulness in presents, "Gifts" could be their love language.

WORDS OF AFFIRMATION:

If "Words of Affirmation" seem to make them glow, consider these strategies:

Encouraging Words: Observe if your loved one frequently offers words of encouragement, praise, or affirmation to others. If they are quick to speak kind and uplifting words, it's a sign that this might be their love language.

Verbal Appreciation: Take note of how they respond to verbal expressions of love and appreciation.

If they cherish compliments, sweet notes, and verbal affection, they are likely receptive to this love language.

Positive Communication: Gauge their preference for positive communication. Do they focus on affirming words and expressions that boost others' self-esteem? If so, "Words of Affirmation" may be their love language.

QUALITY TIME:

Maybe "Quality Time" is what gives them lots of satisfaction. Look for these indicators:

Seek your undivided attention: If quality time is your loved one's love language, they value moments where they have your full, undistracted presence. Be prepared to focus solely on them without distractions.

Enjoy deep conversations: Quality time lovers appreciate meaningful discussions exploring emotions, dreams, and personal experiences.

Value quality over quantity: They prioritize the quality of moments shared rather than the quantity of time spent together. Celebrating milestones together is essential for them.

PHYSICAL TOUCH:

Perhaps your loved one's love language is "Physical Touch"

Responsive Touch: Pay attention to how they respond to physical touch. If they enjoy hugs, kisses, and holding hands, it clearly indicates that physical touch is essential to them.

Comfort in Proximity: Observe their comfort level with close physical proximity. If they prefer sitting closely, leaning in, or seeking physical connection, it's a strong sign that "Physical Touch" is their love language.

Receptive Body Language: Look for positive body language cues when you offer physical affection. If they smile, relax, or show contentment, it indicates they appreciate this love language.

ACTS OF SERVICE:

To discern if your loved one's love language is "Acts of Service," consider these tactics:

Reciprocal Acts: Notice if your loved one often reciprocates acts of service. If they willingly help others and feel fulfilled when others assist them, this is a good sign.

Helping Hand: Observe their willingness to help and support others, especially through actions. If they're the first to lend a hand or offer assistance, "Acts of Service" could be their love language.

Valuing Assistance: Pay attention to how they react when you perform acts of service for them. If they express gratitude, affection, or appreciation for your assistance, it shows the importance of this love language to them.

Keep This in Mind as You Continue on Your Caregiving Journey:

Remember, God IS Love and Love is the fuel that powers your journey. Pour it out generously, and you'll find that it multiplies in the most extraordinary ways.

The insights shared here can help you discover your loved one's primary love language and enhance your caregiving approach to better meet their emotional needs.

Scriptures tell us that God's way is perfect. When we trust in Him, His presence fills us with a deep sense of joy. Trust in God's perfect way in your caregiving journey. It's like having an infallible compass, always leading you in the right direction.

Questions for Reflection:

1. How can you express love through actions in your caregiving role today?
2. How can you discover and understand the love language of your loved one in caregiving?
3. How can you incorporate their love language into your caregiving routine to build trust and strengthen your connection?

Closing Prayer:

Dear Lord, guide us in understanding and embracing the love languages of those we care for. Help us express love in ways that resonate with their hearts, building trust and deepening our connections. May our caregiving journey be filled with the beauty of love and understanding. In Jesus name, we pray. Amen.

Affirmation:

"I embrace the beautiful diversity of love languages, knowing that by understanding and speaking them, I am strengthening the bonds of trust and connection in my caregiving journey."

Your Thoughts:

Day 2: Discovering Love Languages

"You make known to me the path of life; you will fill me with joy in your presence, with eternal pleasures at your right hand." - 2 Samuel 22:31

Welcome to Day 2 of our caregiving journey, where we will continue to delve into the art of understanding and speaking the unique love languages of our loved ones. As we explore this beautiful tapestry of love, we will continually place our trust in God, knowing that His way is perfect.

Just as every artist has a distinct style, every person has a unique love language. And as caregivers, we're about to become experts in decoding these artistic expressions of love.

When you offer love in the way that resonates most deeply with your loved one, you're communicating, "I see you, I hear you, and I love you." It's a beautiful form of connection and the embodiment of the selfless love that Jesus taught.

"Love is the universal language
that transcends countries, borders, barriers, and differences."
- Susan C. Young

Practical Applications:

1. **Observe to Understand:** As we embark on this exploration, remember that observing is the first step to understanding. Take notice of the love clues your loved one leaves. Are they the givers of gifts, expressing their love through tokens of affection? Do their words flow with affirmations, uplifting and reassuring others? By observing their actions and reactions, we can unveil the language of their hearts.

2. **Listen to Their Heartfelt Whispers:** If your loved one desires more quality time together, it's an invitation to open your heart to them. By sharing more of your time, you acknowledge their longing for a deeper connection.

3. **Try on Conversations That Touch the Soul:** Conversations can be the bridge to understanding your loved one's deepest desires. Engage in heartfelt discussions that reveal their joys, fears, and desires. Ask open-ended questions like, "What makes you feel loved and appreciated?" Be an attentive listener. Plan a meaningful conversation with your loved one. Ask them questions about what brings them joy and how you can make them feel cherished. If it's Words of Affirmation seem to resonate, share compliments and words of encouragement with them.

4. **Give Attendance to Their Joys:** The little things that make them happy provide profound insights. Acts of service can light up their day, making them feel loved and cherished.

5. **Experiment with Touch:** For caregivers, touch is a part of the daily routine, yet not all touches are the same. The touch that speaks their love language is one that makes them lean in, smile, and feel content. On the other hand, if they tense up, pull away, or express discomfort, they may be averse to physical touch. Learn to read their cues and understand their comfort zones.

6. **Revive Cherished Memories:** The past holds treasures of their joys and what makes them feel loved. Think back to moments when they were particularly happy or touched by something you or someone else did. These instances are like love language signposts.

7. **Keep Experimenting:** Don't shy away from trying various expressions of love. Experiment with different ways of showing your love. In one week, focus on acts of service, and in another, offer words of affirmation. Their response will reveal their preferred love language.

8. **Collect Love Insights:** Family and friends who have shared in their life journey may offer valuable insights. Discover the heartwarming memories they've created together and relive those beautiful moments.

9. **Exercise Patience:** Understanding a love language is akin to piecing together a puzzle. It requires time and patience. Enjoy this adventure of love, knowing that each piece brings you closer to the complete picture of their heart

10. **Dedicate Time to Activities**: Other interests may be related to your loved one's apparent love language. What type of activities were enjoyed in the past

11. **Take Moments to Consider:** There are always moments in the past that brought happiness to your

loved one, so consider how these instances may reveal their prevalent love language.

As you explore these unique languages of love, remember that your caregiving journey is a beautiful tapestry of selfless love. As we continue our caregiving journey, remember that understanding and speaking your loved one's love language is a profound way to demonstrate your care and devotion. With patience and attentive observation, you can build a deeper connection and create moments filled with love and understanding.

Questions for Reflection:

1. How have you observed your loved one's love language clues?
2. What do you think your loved one's love language might be?
3. What heartfelt conversations have you engaged in recently?
4. Can you recall moments when your loved one lights up with joy?

Closing Prayer:

Dear Lord, as we embark on this journey of learning and discovering Love Languages, we trust that You will guide us, empower us, and fill our hearts with the boundless love that transcends language. Please help us to minister Your Unconditional Love we care for our loved ones.

Your Thoughts:

Day 3: Never-Ending Housework

FINDING BALANCE AMID CHORES

"Come to me, all you who are weary and burdened, and I will give you rest." - Matthew 11:28

Welcome back, caregivers, to Day 3 of our adventure. Today, we're tackling a universal caregiver challenge – piles of laundry, dishes in the sink, and stuff strewn throughout the house. It often feels like being caught in a whirlwind, hedged in by all the activities of daily living. But remember that balance is the key, and rest is your best friend.

Matthew 11:28 extends a comforting invitation from Jesus himself. It's as though He's calling out, saying, "Yoo Hoo (your name), yes you, my beloved, the one I love, the one feeling lost in the sauce – Come, rest, and leave that concoction of chores for a while. Take a break." Now, picture yourself amid life's tornado, trading the pressure you feel for the comfort of sinking into a soft, cozy lounge chair. Before settling into the chair, you cast aside your thoughts and cares, placing them into the loving embrace of your Heavenly Father's arms. After you've entrusted the whirlwind of thoughts and cares to Him, experience the deep rest He provides.

So much demands attention. It's so important for us to maintain both an emotional and physical balance amid all the various tasks we have to manage. Sometimes, it feels like we're walking a tightrope.

Speaking of balance, Rumi, the ancient poet, knew the dance between holding on and letting go all too well. Caregiving teaches us that sometimes we must let go of what we can't control and hold on to our sanity. It's a delicate act, but trust me, God will show you the moves to stabilize your footing.

Oh, and don't forget this. As you whirl among the flurry of household chores, laundry, and caregiving duties, find a reason to smile – it will smooth out all the wrinkles!

> "Life is a balance of holding on and letting go."
> Rumi

> "Balance, like a tightrope walker, is not about never losing your balance; it's about finding it again."
> Linda Poindexter

Practical Applications:

1. Mindful Moments on the Move: Turn routine tasks into opportunities for mental calmness. While you go about your daily chores, practice deep breathing and positive affirmations, or visualize a tranquil scene with Jesus right beside you. These mindfulness techniques can help soothe your mind while in motion, making the most of your caregiving moments. You might like to memorize and meditate on a scripture verse while folding a mountain of

laundry. This will get The Word into your spirit so it will be right there inside of you when you need it in the future. You can also take some time while moving here and there from task to task to listen to a podcast or YouTube video about whatever tickles your fancy at the time. The most important thing is for you to find rest in your labor as you enter into His Rest.

2. Ask for Help: Don't be shy about asking for a helping hand. Caregiving doesn't mean you have to do it all alone. Delegate tasks and share the workload. If you have no one readily available to share responsibilities with, you can turn to Abba Father in prayer and ask Him to send a willing helper.

3. Take Time to do something that brings you peace. Be mindful that whatever you do is in God's Presence. When you are doing something (or nothing) that makes you feel good and relaxed, that's a good thing. Dedicate at least 15 minutes each day just for you. Can you do that? Sip a cup of tea, read a few pages of a book, take a quick cat nap *set the alarm on your cell phone if you're afraid of oversleeping*, close your eyes, sigh, breathe, whatever floats your boat at the time. It will be a mini-vacation for your soul.

Questions for Reflection

1. How can you find moments of rest and relaxation amid your caregiving responsibilities?
2. What can you let go of today that's been adding unnecessary weight to your already busy life?

Closing Prayer:

Heavenly Father, in the middle of these never-ending chores, piles of laundry, and caregiving craziness, grant us the wisdom to find balance. Remind us to take a break when we're weary and to let go of what's beyond our control. Be our source of rest and strength. In Jesus Name Amen.

Affirmation:

I find balance and rest in the midst of life's whirlwind.

Your Thoughts:

Day 4: Crisis Mode

FINDING CALM IN THE STORM

"When you pass through the waters, I will be with you; and when you pass through the rivers, they will not sweep over you. When you walk through the fire, you will not be burned; the flames will not set you ablaze." - Isaiah 43:2

Hello and welcome to Day 4 of our journey. Today, we're exploring how to find calm in the middle of life's storms. Isaiah 43:2 extends a comforting promise that carries a profound message for caregivers facing trying and tumultuous times. Remember, as we walk through the rough waters and fiery trials of life, God is with us. Even though we may not see Him with our physical eyes, we can perceive His presence with our spiritual vision. God accompanies us through waves of uncertainty. God's Word encourages us to rely on the inner strength that God provides. His Word fortifies our faith, enabling us to withstand the emotional and spiritual trials we encounter. By embracing faith, we are practicing patience. This makes us more resilient and ultimately brings us inner peace. In the heart of the storm that you discover your true strength.

"In the middle of every difficulty lies opportunity."
- Albert Einstein

Practical Applications:

1. **In your spare time** (which there probably isn't much of), **Create a mental "emergency kit"** stocked with positive affirmations. This way, when the storm rages, and you feel yourself sinking into despair, open that kit and let those affirmations be your anchor.
2. **Look Through a Different Lens:** Train yourself to see opportunities within difficulties. Ask yourself, "What can I learn from this situation?" or "In what way can I find calm in the midst of chaos?" Seek to see your predicament from a perfect right angle.
3. **Trust Resilience:** Trust God's Goodness. Also, remind yourself of past hurdles you've overcome. Know that you have the inner strength and stamina to make it through the storm.
4. **Praise the Lord:** Let His Word be in your mouth. Remember that God inhabits the praises of His people. Praise brings His Power into the scene.

Questions for Reflection:

1. How can you tap into God's presence and assurance when you find yourself in crisis mode during your caregiving journey?
2. Recall a recent crisis you faced. What opportunities for growth and compassion did it present?
3. Can you identify a time when you felt the presence of God during a personal storm?

Closing Prayer:

Heavenly Father, in the midst of life's storms, we often feel overwhelmed and uncertain. Yet, we find solace in the knowledge that You are our anchor, our refuge. Help us to find calm amidst the chaos and recognize the opportunities that difficulties bring. Guide us through every crisis, for with You by our side, we are never alone. In Jesus' name, we pray. Amen.

Affirmation:

"I am resilient, guided by faith, and strengthened through challenges. With God's presence, I find calm in the midst of life's storms."

Your Thoughts:

Day 5: Navigating Emotional Storms

FINDING PEACE AND LIBERATING LOVE FROM GUILT

"Do not be anxious about anything, but in every situation, by prayer and petition, with thanksgiving, present your requests to God. And the peace of God, which transcends all understanding, will guard your hearts and your minds in Christ Jesus." - Philippians 4:6-7

Caregivers, you are welcome to Day 5. Today, we're delving into the depths of emotional storms, where even the strongest swimmers can feel overwhelmed. But take heart; you're not riding this sea of emotions alone.

God knows exactly how you feel, and He's with you every step of the way. So, let's embark on a voyage to find peace amid the chaos of emotional stress.

Philippians 4:6-7 encourages us not to be anxious but to bring our concerns to God through prayer and thanksgiving. In return, God's peace, a peace beyond human understanding, stands guard over our hearts and minds. It's like having a divine emotional lifebuoy to keep you afloat.

As a child, I often grappled with overwhelming feelings of guilt. My happiness seemed intricately tied to my mother's, and I believed that if she was happy, I could be happy too. This childhood pattern haunted me, leaving a legacy of guilt that extended into my adult life and affected my intimate relationships. The belief that I was responsible for my mother's happiness led to a lifelong struggle with codependency.

I discovered that I was prone to people-pleasing behaviors, always striving to do more and be more to ensure my mother's happiness. Even when I wasn't the cause of her distress, I felt guilty and would make relentless efforts to bring her joy. This pattern of behavior contributed to the development of codependency in my life, becoming a stronghold that took years to break free from.

My journey towards recovery from codependency was a lengthy one, but it was during the 13 years I cared for my mother until her passing at the age of 94 that I truly began to identify and confront the traits of codependency. This experience compelled me to ensure that my caregiving was driven not by guilt but by genuine love, compassion, and authenticity.

Today, we're looking into the critical theme of liberating love from the grip of guilt. In caregiving, it's crucial to examine our motives.

Childhood experiences can sometimes leave us shackled by guilt, leading to people-pleasing behaviors that persist into adulthood. We may feel responsible for the happiness of our loved ones, even when their well-being isn't within our control.

Caregiving should flow from the pure love that originates from the heart of God, not from guilt. We must be aware of the subtle influence of guilt in our caregiving journey and strive to replace it with love, compassion, and authenticity. Remember, you are enough just as you are, and God's love is your guiding light.

"You are not alone on this journey. God knows exactly how you feel, and He's with you every step of the way."
— Unknown

Practical Application:

1. **Seek Truth:** Examine the beliefs and mental patterns that trigger guilt. Accept the truth that you are loved and valued by God, regardless of your actions.
2. **Set Healthy Boundaries:** Recognize that you cannot control the happiness of others. Set healthy boundaries that protect your emotional well-being while still providing love and care.
3. **Embrace Self-Love:** Practice self-love and self-compassion. Remember that your worth is not determined by the happiness of others.
4. **Choose Love over Guilt:** Make decisions and take actions that are rooted in love rather than guilt.
5. **Talk It Out:** Don't bottle up your emotions. Talk to a friend, a family member, or a support group about what you're going through. Sometimes, just sharing the load can lighten the emotional burden.
6. **Take a moment to reflect** on how the idea of releasing guilt and embracing love resonates with you. When emotional stress hits, take a moment not only to talk to God, but also to listen for the still small voice of Love. Pour out your feelings, fears, and frustrations to God. He's always there to listen. How will you apply this perspective in your caregiving journey? Share your thoughts and experiences.

Questions for Reflection:

1. Take a moment to reflect on your caregiving journey. Have feelings of guilt influenced your actions? How can you release guilt and embrace love instead?
2. What steps can you take to ensure that your caregiving is driven by love and authenticity, rather than the need for affirmation?
3. Are you driven by a sincere desire to care for your loved one, or are guilt and the need for affirmation guiding your actions?
4. Have you felt the presence of God in your caregiving journey?
5. How does God's presence in your life liberate you from the chains of guilt in your caregiving journey.

Closing Prayer:

Fill us with your pure love and guide us to care for our loved ones from a place of authenticity and compassion. Teach us to bring our worries to You, to express our gratitude even in trying times, and to lean on the support of others. Guard our hearts and minds with Your transcendent peace. In Jesus' Name, we pray. Amen.

Affirmation:

"I choose to release guilt and embrace love in my caregiving journey. With God's guidance, I find peace amid the emotional storms."

Your Thoughts:

Day 6: Finding Energy in the Midst of Demands

YOUR OWN WELL-BEING FRONT AND CENTER

"But those who hope in the LORD will renew their strength. They will soar on wings like eagles; they will run and not grow weary, they will walk and not be faint." - Isaiah 40:31

Hello, dear caregivers, and welcome to Day 6 of our journey. Today, we're addressing the physical demands and exhaustion often accompanying caregiving. Sometimes It's like running a marathon with no finish line in sight. But remember, even marathon runners need to catch their breath.

Scripture reminds us that those who hope in the Lord will renew their strength. It's like a promise of energy, resilience, and endurance. When you feel like you're running on empty, God is your source of renewal.

As a family caregiver, it's natural for the needs of your loved one to be in the forefront of your attention. However, today, we're placing a spotlight on your own well-being, bringing it front and center. Just as a car requires regular maintenance to run smoothly, you also need self-care to maintain your caregiving journey effectively.

Don't worry about resting when you're weary. It's not a sign of weakness; it's a necessity. If you get enough rest, you're more likely to recover quickly. Even short catnaps can do you a world of good. Even Jesus needed a break.

"Rest when you're weary. Refresh and renew yourself, your body, your mind, your spirit. Then get back to work"
- Ralph Marston

"Taking care of yourself doesn't mean me first, it means me too."
- L.R. Knost

Practical Applications:

1. Embrace Power Naps: Allow yourself short power naps during the day. Fifteen to twenty minutes can work wonders to refresh your energy.
2. Ask for Help: Don't be shy about asking for a helping hand. Caregiving doesn't mean you have to do it all alone. Delegate tasks and share the load. Hopefully, there is somebody around to delegate to, but if not,, perhaps getting someone to come in for just a few hours here and there will do wonders to rejuvenate you.
3. Set Boundaries: Establish clear boundaries for your caregiving responsibilities. Know when it's time to say no to additional tasks or commitments.
4. Respite Care: Investigate care services in your area and familiarize what Adult Day Care programs are available in your area. Enrolling your loved one in a

social or medical adult daycare program is an excellent way to get some time for yourself. It is also good for your loved one.

Questions for Reflection:

1. How can you incorporate short breaks and moments of rest into your daily caregiving routine?
2. Are there any caregiving tasks that you can delegate or share with others to lighten your physical load?

Closing Prayer:

Heavenly Father, in the midst of physical demands and exhaustion, we sometimes feel drained. But we remember that in You, we find renewal and strength. Teach us to rest when we're weary, to seek help when needed, and to set boundaries to protect our well-being. Grant us the endurance to continue this caregiving journey. In Jesus Name Amen.

Affirmation:

"I am worthy of love and care for myself. My well-being matters.

Your Thoughts:

Day 7: Mastering Time

FINDING MOMENTS OF CLARITY IN THE CHAOS

"Teach us to number our days, that we may gain a heart of wisdom." - Psalm 90:12 (NIV)

Hello again, wonderful caregivers, and welcome to Day 7 of our journey. Today, we're exploring the art of time management – a skill that can sometimes feel as elusive as chasing fireflies in the night. But fear not, you can do it.

Psalm 90:12 invites us to "number our days" – to recognize the preciousness of time. In the whirlwind of caregiving, it's easy to lose track, but every moment counts. Wisdom lies in how we spend those moments.

And speaking of wisdom, Michael Altshuler gives us a little gem – time flies, but you're the pilot. Picture yourself in the cockpit, steering through the skies of your day. You have the controls, even when time is flying away from you.

One of my life's goals was to learn to fly. I thought I'd get a chance at that and maybe even get my pilot license when I lived in Austin, Texas back in the 70's. I was a Nurse Paramedic for the City in those days and I worked with several guys who were pilots. One of my EMS buddies, a flight instructor, offered to train me for free. I sure wanted to take a crack at that and take him up on the offer, but for some reason, can't remember why now, I never got around to it. I'm not particularly fond of flying when someone else has the plane's yoke in hand, but flying with me in control…I like that scenario best as long as I was sufficiently trained. Little did I know back then that the chance to fly a plane in the literal sky would pass me by, and little did I know that the kind of flying I'd be doing would be me at the controls of my own life choices.

When I feel confused and losing it I force myself to remember that "this too shall pass."

"The bad news is time flies.
The good news is you're the pilot."
- Michael Altshuler

Practical Applications:

1. Create a Daily Routine: Craft a daily schedule that allocates specific time for caregiving tasks, self-care, and moments of relaxation. Stick to it as closely as possible.
2. Prioritize Tasks: Identify the most important caregiving tasks and tackle them first. Remember, not everything needs to be done today. Prioritize what truly matters.
3. Delegate and Seek Support: Don't hesitate to delegate tasks or seek support from friends and family. It takes a village to navigate the caregiving universe

Questions for Reflection:

- What tasks can you delegate or share with others to free up more of your valuable time?
- Can you create a daily routine that balances caregiving responsibilities with self-care and rest?

Closing Prayer:

Heavenly Father, in the midst of the chaotic demands of care-giving, or problems that arise around us we sometimes lose sight of time. We recognize its preciousness and ask for the wisdom to use it wisely. Help us pilot our days with intention and purpose, finding clarity even in the chaos. Thank you for Your loving care and support. In Jesus Name Amen.

Affirmation:

"Even when time seems like quicksilver in my hands, I will remember that I have the power to shape it into something beautiful and meaningful."

Your Thoughts:

Day 8: Juggling Too Many Roles

FINDING HARMONY IN LIFE'S CIRCUS

"Cast your cares on the LORD and he will sustain you; he will never let the righteous be shaken." - Psalm 55:22

Hello, amazing caregivers, and welcome to Day 8 of our adventure. Today, we're diving into the complex art of juggling – not just tasks but roles. It's like being the ringmaster of your own circus, who is also experienced at juggling. Trust me, you've got this show under control even if you don't realize it. However, while we might be the ringmasters of our own little circus, God is still and always will be the Ultimate Ringmaster and juggler. Remember that we will always be the mentee while God is The Grand Mentor. We can trust the Holy Spirit to help us run our show on Earth while God is running the Greatest Show not only on Earth, but the Greatest Show in the Universe!

Psalm 55:22 offers a promise of sustenance when you cast your cares on the Lord. Picture you throwing those juggling balls high into the air, knowing that God's steady hand will catch them. And even if you drop a ball once in a while, it's okay because God is able to make all grace abound toward you.

Life is indeed a circus, with acts upon acts, and you, my dear caregiver, are the ringmaster. Embrace this role with a sense of wonder and curiosity. Keep the show going, even when it feels like you're juggling flaming swords.

> "Life is like a circus. There's always something happening, and you're the ringmaster. Keep the show going!"
> - Unknown

Practical Applications:

1. Prioritize and Delegate: List your roles – caregiver, family member, friend, employee – and prioritize them. Delegate when possible, and don't be afraid to ask for help.
2. Schedule "Me" Time: Dedicate regular slots in your schedule just for yourself. It's essential to recharge your batteries and maintain your inner ringmaster.
3. Lean on Your Support Network: Rely on your support network, whether it's friends, family, or support groups. They can be your safety net when the juggling gets tough.

Questions for Reflection:

1. How can you find harmony and balance between your various roles as a caregiver and in other areas of your life?
2. Are there tasks or responsibilities that you can let go of, or people you can reach out to for support in your juggling act?

Closing Prayer:

Heavenly Father, as we juggle the many roles life has given us, we often feel like circus performers in the center ring. But we know that when we cast our cares on You, we find sustenance and strength. Guide us in finding harmony amid life's chaos and help us keep the show going with grace. With Your guidance we can become expert jugglers. Thank you for helping us catch the ball and run the show. In Jesus Name. Amen

Affirmation:

I can do hard things because God is always with me to help in one way or another.

Your Thoughts:

Day 9: Maneuvering Financial Rapids

KEEPING YOUR HEAD ABOVE WATER

"And my God will meet all your needs according to the riches of his glory in Christ Jesus." - Philippians 4:19

Hello servant-hearted caregivers, and welcome to Day 9 of our incredible journey. Today, we're diving into the financial strains of caregiving – a topic that can feel like navigating treacherous rapids. But fear not, for you have God's unwavering source of strength and love to stabilize you through the ever so bumpy ride.

Philippians 4:19 assures us that God will meet all our needs according to His riches. It's like having a never-ending wellspring of support, even in the face of financial challenges. You may not see the entire staircase, but God provides the next step. You do you best and God will do the rest. You rest and God will do His best to deliver you from the troubles you face. Know that God is on your side and He always has a solution to our problems. Whenever I find myself undergoing financial woes I start sing that "God Will Make A Way." Sung by Don Moen. It always picks me up and lifts me out of fear and confusion. Try it. It works!

Corrie ten Boom wisely reminds us that worrying doesn't empty tomorrow of its sorrow; it empties today of its strength. So, as you navigate the financial rapids of caregiving, trust that your strength, your resilience, and your resourcefulness will guide you.

> "Worrying doesn't empty tomorrow of its sorrow,
> it empties today of its strength."
> - Corrie ten Boom

Practical Applications:

1. Explore Cost-Cutting: Investigate ways to reduce caregiving expenses, such as utilizing community services or seeking discounts for medical supplies.
2. Create a caregiving budget and explore financial resources. There are many resources online to help you
3. Consult a financial advisor or your accountant for professional advice.

Questions for Reflection:

1. How can you proactively address and manage the financial strains associated with caregiving?
2. In what ways can you cultivate peace and resilience in the face of financial challenges?

Closing Prayer:

Heavenly Father, as caregivers facing financial challenges, we sometimes feel overwhelmed. Help us to remember that You are our provider, meeting our needs even in difficult times. Grant us the wisdom to navigate the financial rapids we get caught up in. Help us find peace during the times when financial pressures threaten to drown us. Lead us and guide us to those who can help us understand what we may not know to do or what we need to do to help ourselves to a better place. Thank you In Jesus Name Amen.

Affirmation:

"I've got what it takes to navigate this journey. I will remember that even in turbulent financial times, my greatest assets are resourcefulness and resilience."

Your Thoughts:

Day 10: Balancing Act Mastery

SPINNING WORK AND CAREGIVING PLATES WITH POISE

"But he said to me, 'My grace is sufficient for you, for my power is made perfect in weakness.'" - 2 Corinthians 12:9

Hi Working Caregivers! Today, we're going to focus on the delicate balance between work and caregiving because so many are handling outside jobs and caregiving for their loved ones at the same time. This can become more and more taxing on the soul due to the substantial hardship that arises when attempting to excel in both areas. It seems like we need to emulate the expertise of a plate-spinning performer, ensuring each plate continues to spin until the moment we choose to stop. In the delicate interplay of caregiving and work, always remember that companionship surrounds you. Share your thoughts and experiences with others encountering similar challenges, and allow the encouragement from your faith community and loved ones to fortify you in this intricate balancing act. Together, we will discover the strength and grace needed to traverse these life complexities. Let us consider practical solutions that can make this intricate dance more manageable. In the rapidly evolving work landscape of today, exploring options such as remote work, flexible hours, or even job sharing can provide the flexibility needed to fulfill caregiving duties while remaining committed to our professional responsibilities. Lord knows some people need their paycheck. In my own case, I left shift work in favor of making my own hours and successfully transitioned into the field of RN Care Management, Concierge Nursing, and Patient Advocacy. In this win-win situation, both my clients and I reap the benefits. They draw from my 50 years of professional nursing expertise, and I get to do what I like best. I also took on Geriatric clients who needed Elder and Medical Massage. This Ministry of Health is right up my alley.

So, that's how both ends met for me. Now, how can both ends meet for you if this balancing act is or becomes more unbearable?

"Believe you can and you're halfway there."
- Theodore Roosevelt

Practical Applications:

1. Prioritize Tasks: Identify and prioritize tasks at work and in caregiving, focusing on the most critical aspects to maintain balance.
2. Effective Communication: Have open and honest conversations with both your employer and your loved one about your situation, seeking understanding and support.
3. Explore Flexible Work Arrangements: a. Remote Work: For jobs that allow it, explore the possibility of working remotely, providing flexibility to fulfill caregiving duties while maintaining productivity. b. Flexible Hours: Work with your employer to establish flexible working hours, enabling you to accommodate

caregiving responsibilities without compromising work quality. c. Job Sharing: Investigate the potential for job sharing, where responsibilities and hours are divided between two employees, ensuring the work is covered while providing the caregiver with needed flexibility.

Questions for Reflection:

1. How can you lean on God's grace to find strength in the midst of the balancing act between work and caregiving?
2. In what ways can effective communication with your employer and loved one alleviate the challenges you face?
3. Have you explored all available options for flexible work arrangements to better manage your caregiving responsibilities?

Closing Prayer:

Gracious Father, in the midst of the delicate dance between work and caregiving, we seek Your wisdom and strength. Grant us the grace to navigate this balancing act with resilience and love. May our efforts bring glory to Your name. In Jesus' name, we pray. Amen.

Affirmations:

"I am resilient and capable of navigating the challenges of balancing work and caregiving. God's grace empowers me to fulfill my responsibilities with love and dedication."

Your Thoughts:

Day 11: Surrender for Serenity

LET GO AND FORGIVE FOR THE HEALTH OF IT

"Bear with each other and forgive one another if any of you has a grievance against someone. Forgive as the Lord forgave you." - Colossians 3:13

Hello, beloved caregiver. Today, I want to talk to you about a topic that may be very difficult for some of you: forgiveness. Forgiveness is not easy, especially when you have been hurt by the people who are supposed to love and support you. You may have experienced betrayal, rejection, criticism, gossip, or even hostility from your relatives or friends because of your decision to care for your loved one. You may feel angry, hurt, bitter, or resentful towards them. You may wonder how they can be so selfish, insensitive, or cruel. You may feel like you have no one to turn to or trust.

If this is you, I understand how you feel. I have been in your shoes. I am a family caregiver myself and have experienced what it is like to be treated with disdain by those I never expected it from. Our loved one asked me to be her primary caregiver and to let her move in with us. Let me be clear, I did not ask her, she asked us. When she realized she could no longer live alone in her own home without 24/7 care and help and refused to have someone who wasn't family or already her friend come live with her she shifted gears. She became emphatic about "absolutely" not wanting to go to a nursing home or assisted living facility. Even though I tried my best to convince her how great this option would be for her she kept saying, "Nope, not for me." I took her to no less than 12 AL places, but she was against it. Then she asked if we'd let her come live with us. We thought it over and said, "Yes." That's when all hell broke loose.

She already had entrusted me as her medical power of attorney partly because I am a Registered Nurse who specializes in dementia care and Geriatric Care Management, but this was a BIG STEP beyond.

Not everyone in our extended family was happy with her choice. I was accused of conniving and talking her into staying with us. If that was my schtick, why then did I take her to visit other places for a few years already? One of those beloved relatives, convinced I was in it for the money, screamed "Scam Artist" at me from across the street so our neighbors could hear. Wow…that was quite an eye and ear-opener! And guess who saw this happen? You got it. Our loved one who was watching it occur because she was standing at the front door looking out at the scene. There were those who wanted her to go to a facility. They said they would visit her there, but if she lived with us, they would no longer visit her. Lies, accusations, and rumors were spread about me. Somebody even reported me to Adult Protective Services to ruin my excellent professional reputation, but it didn't work the way they'd hoped. Instead, the APS worker saw it as the "typical family stunt" they see all the time from disgruntled relatives.

Their actions against me made my life very difficult and stressful. I was hurt very deeply by the ones I love; however, I did not let the pain of it stick. I did not let them rob me of the joy and peace that I have in caring for our loved one. I did not let them ruin my relationship with God or with her. I did not let them make me bitter or hateful. I chose to forgive them and to let go and let God take care of things while I continued to do what I was called by God to do.

Why did I forgive them? Because I love God and that's what God tells us to do if we profess to love him. Because God commands me to forgive others as He forgave me. Because God's Holy Spirit gives me the grace and the strength to forgive. Because forgiveness is good for me and for them as well. Because forgiveness sets me free from the bondage of anger and resentment. Because forgiveness heals me and restores me. Because forgiveness honors God and glorifies Him. And most of all because we Christians are to make Love our greatest aim.

How did I forgive them? By following the example of Jesus, who forgave those who crucified Him. By praying for them and blessing them. By letting go of the past and focusing on the present. By refusing to retaliate or seek revenge. By speaking the truth in love and seeking reconciliation. By trusting God to judge them and vindicate me. By remembering that they are also human and sinful, and that they need God's mercy and grace. By realizing that they do not know what they are doing, and that they are hurting themselves more than they are hurting me.

Forgiveness is not easy, but it is possible. Forgiveness is not a one-time event, but a continuous process. Forgiveness is not a feeling, but a choice. Forgiveness is not a weakness, but a strength. Forgiveness is not a burden, but a blessing.

I encourage you to forgive those who hurt you. I know it is hard, but it is worth it. You will feel lighter, happier, and healthier. You will experience God's love, peace, and joy. You will grow closer to God and to your loved one. You will be a better caregiver and a better person.

> "To forgive is to set a prisoner free and discover that the prisoner was you."
> - Lewis B. Smedes

Practical Applications:

Identify the people who have hurt you because of your caregiving role. Write down their names and what they did or said to you. Then write down how you feel about them and how you have reacted to them.

1. Pray for each person on your list. Ask God to forgive them and to bless them. Ask God to forgive you and to heal you. Ask God to help you forgive them and to release them from your anger and resentment. Ask God to give you His perspective and His grace. Ask God to show you how to love them and to deal with them in a godly way.

2. Take action to demonstrate your forgiveness. This may include sending them a card, a gift, or a message of love and appreciation. It may also include inviting them to visit your loved one, or to join you for a meal or a coffee. It may also include confronting them in a respectful and honest manner, and expressing your feelings and your expectations. It may also include seeking professional help or legal advice if necessary. Do whatever you feel led by God to do, but do it in a spirit of love and peace.

Questions for Reflection:

Why is forgiveness important for you as a caregiver?

1. What are the benefits of forgiving those who hurt you?
2. What are the challenges or obstacles that prevent you from forgiving them?
3. How can you overcome these challenges or obstacles?
4. How do you know that you have truly forgiven them?

Closing Prayer:

Dear Heavenly Father, thank You for Your forgiveness and Your love. Thank You for sending Your Son Jesus to die for me and to forgive me. Thank You for giving me the opportunity to care for my loved one and to serve You. I confess that I have been hurt by some people who do not understand or appreciate my caregiving role. I confess that I have been angry, bitter, or resentful towards them. I confess that I have not forgiven them as You have forgiven me. Please forgive me, Lord, and cleanse me from all unrighteousness. Please heal me from all the wounds and scars that they have inflicted on me. Please fill me with Your Holy Spirit and Your grace. Please help me to forgive them and to release them from my heart. Please help me to love them and to bless them. Please help me to seek Your will and Your glory in all my relationships. Please protect me and my loved one from any harm or evil that may come from them. Please restore and reconcile us if it is possible and if it is Your desire. Please make me a peacemaker and a bridge-builder. Please make me a reflection of Your forgiveness and Your love. In Jesus' name, I pray. Amen.

Affirmations:

I am a forgiven and forgiving person. I forgive others as God forgives me. I choose to let go of the past and to embrace the present. I choose to love and bless those who hurt me. I choose to trust God and to follow His guidance. I choose to live in peace and joy.

Your Thoughts:

Day 12: Reconnecting in Isolation

"A friend loves at all times, and a brother is born for a time of adversity." - Proverbs 17:17

Greetings, beloved caregivers! As we embark on this devotional journey together, may you find solace in the warmth of friendship and the comfort of God's presence.

In times of isolation, reaching out to friends may seem like a small act, but it can have a profound impact on our well-being. As caregivers, let's embrace the support that friendships offer, recognizing that we don't walk this journey alone. Share your thoughts and experiences with those around you, and let the bonds of friendship strengthen your spirit.

"A real friend is one who walks in when the rest
of the world walks out."
- Walter Winchell

Practical Applications:

Schedule Virtual Gatherings: Set regular virtual meet-ups with friends through video calls or online platforms to bridge the physical distance.

1. **Share Prayer Requests:** Openly share your concerns and joys with trusted friends, allowing them to join you in prayer and support.
2. **Send Thoughtful Messages:** Take a few moments each day to send encouraging messages or uplifting scriptures to friends, fostering a sense of connection.

Questions for Reflection:

How have your friendships supported you during challenging times?

1. In what ways can you intentionally nurture your friendships despite physical separation?
2. Have you considered seeking support from friends, sharing the responsibilities of caregiving?

Closing Prayer:

Dear Heavenly Father, we come before you with gratitude for the gift of friendship. In this season of caregiving and isolation, may we find strength in our connections with others. Bless our efforts to nurture friendships from afar, and may your love bind us together. In Jesus' name, we pray. Amen.

Affirmations:

"I am surrounded by the love of friends, near and far. In the midst of isolation, my heart is connected to a community that uplifts and supports me."

Your Thoughts:

Day 13: Navigating the Wilderness

WHEN SUPPORT FALTERS

"I can do all this through him who gives me strength." - Philippians 4:13

Hello, dear caregivers, and welcome to a crucial discussion. Today, we're exploring a challenge many caregivers face – the unexpected absence of support from family and friends. It's like embarking on a journey with a map leading to uncharted territory, finding yourself alone as others who were once on this journey with you drop out. Yet, as a caregiver, you're not truly alone. God is there to comfort, guide, and protect you along the path of righteousness in the wilderness.

In my caregiving journey, I've encountered moments of isolation where the support I expected seemed to vanish. I've gone to my own church community asking for help from some of the outreach groups that my church promotes, but the only one I can get any help from is the prayer ministry. What I am saying here is that there really don't seem to be many churches that outreach to people...can I say... in our predicament? And I do mean predicament as in a difficult situation. While this scenario can be disheartening, I am heartened by knowing that God is faithful, His support is unwavering, and He will never forsake us or leave us desolate.

"Sometimes the strongest people are the ones who love beyond all faults, cry behind closed doors, and fight battles that nobody knows about."
- Albert Schweitzer

Practical Applications:

1. **Seek Alternative Support:** Explore local caregiver support groups, and online communities. You can also ask for help from a parachurch outreach groups. Each of these options are places where you can connect with others who understand your journey.
2. **Communicate Your Needs:** Have open and honest conversations with family and friends about your caregiving challenges. They might not be aware of the support you require. After doing this and still not getting the support you think you need, keep your mind fixed on Jesus, the Author and Finisher of Your Faith.
3. **Prioritize Self-Care:** In the absence of expected support, prioritize self-care. Take moments for yourself, rest, and recharge.

Questions for Reflection:

1. **Assess Your Support System:** Reflect on your current support system. Who has been a consistent source of support, and how can you strengthen those connections?
2. **Communicating Expectations**: Have you clearly communicated your needs and expectations to your

family and friends? How can you express your requirements more effectively?

3. **Personal Resilience:** In the absence of expected support, how can you build resilience within yourself? What practices bring you comfort and strength?.

Closing Prayer:

Heavenly Father, as we navigate the wilderness of caregiving, we sometimes feel alone. In these moments, remind us of your constant presence. Strengthen us with the assurance that, through Christ, we can endure and find the support we need. Guide us, Lord, in the paths of righteousness, and let us feel your comforting presence. In Jesus' name, we pray. Amen.

Affirmation:

I am not alone in my caregiving journey. God's strength is my constant companion, and I can navigate the challenges with His unwavering support.

Your Thoughts:

Day 14: Deciphering the Medical Puzzle

FINDING CLARITY AMID COMPLEXITY AND A VOICE OF REASON IN A SEA OF MEDICAL JARGON

"Trust in the LORD with all your heart and lean not on your own understanding; in all your ways submit to him, and he will make your paths straight." - Proverbs 3:5-6

Hello, resilient caregivers, and welcome to Day Thirteen of our incredible journey. Today, we're diving into a complex topic – deciphering medical jargon and confronting intricate medical issues. It's like trying to solve a puzzle but remember, you have the pieces within you.

Proverbs 3:5-6 advises us to trust in the Lord with all our hearts and lean not on our understanding. In moments of medical complexity, it's essential to submit to a higher power and trust that the path will become clear.

In every problem, there's a hidden solution waiting to be found. Think of it as a treasure hunt – you're on a quest for answers and clarity. Each medical issue you face brings you closer to understanding and wisdom.

And remember caregivers, you are like detectives in the world of healthcare, searching for clues and solutions to ensure the best care for your loved one. Each step you take brings you closer to understanding the complete picture.

> "In every problem, there's a hidden solution
> just waiting to be found."
> - Unknown

Practical Applications:

1. Ask Questions: Don't hesitate to ask your medical team questions until you fully understand the situation, treatment options, and potential outcomes.
2. Seek Second Opinions: If you're unsure about a diagnosis or treatment plan, consider seeking a second opinion from another medical professional.
3. Educate Yourself: Empower yourself with knowledge by researching your loved one's condition and treatment options. Just ensure your sources are reputable.

Questions for Reflection:

1. How can you effectively communicate with your medical team to gain a better understanding of complex medical issues?
2. Are there additional resources or experts you can consult to navigate the intricacies of your loved one's medical condition?

Closing Prayer:

Heavenly Father, when we're confronted with complex medical issues, we may feel lost in a sea of uncertainty. But we trust in Your guidance and wisdom. Help us ask the right questions, seek second opinions, and educate ourselves to find clarity amid complexity. In Jesus Name Amen.

Affirmations:

I trust in the Lord with all my heart and seek wisdom as I confront complex medical issues. Like a diligent detective, I see each challenge as a puzzle to be solved, discovering hidden solutions with faith and determination. I confidently ask questions, seek second opinions, and educate myself, drawing closer to understanding and clarity in the world of medical intricacies.

Your Thoughts:

Day 15: Guided by the North Star

LEARNING TO LIVE IN AN UNSCRIPTED ROLE

"If any of you lacks wisdom, you should ask God, who gives generously to all without finding fault, and it will be given to you. But when you ask, you must believe and not doubt, because the one who doubts is like a wave of the sea, blown and tossed by the wind. That person should not expect to receive anything from the Lord." - James 1:5-7

Hello, Bright and Shining Caregivers. God's light is shining on you even if you don't feel it. Welcome to Day 15 of our heartwarming journey. Today, we're exploring a role that many of you didn't train for – the role of a doctor or nurse, suddenly thrust upon you. It's like being handed a script for a play you never auditioned for, but remember, you're the star of this show.

We, as caregivers, shine as stars in our roles, finding strength not only in our capabilities but also in the guidance of our divine North Star, God, the most magnificent star of all.

Philippians 4:13 reminds us that we can do all things through him who strengthens us. When you find yourself in a care-giving role you never expected, know that you're not alone.

God is your guiding light. In many indigenous cultures, the North Star was seen as a symbol of the Great Spirit, guiding the people on their journey through life. Let's agree that the North Star remains that same meaningful symbol of guidance and direction for us too.

"Believe you can and you're halfway there."
- Theodore Roosevelt

Practical Applications:

1. **Seek Training:** If possible, explore caregiver training programs or resources that can help you gain the skills and knowledge needed for your caregiving role.
2. **Lean on Professionals:** Don't hesitate to consult healthcare professionals for guidance and support. They can provide valuable insights and advice.
3. **Self-Care:** Prioritize self-care to ensure you have the physical and emotional strength to fulfill your caregiving responsibilities.

Questions for Reflection:

1. How can you embrace your caregiving role with openness and a willingness to learn, even when it feels overwhelming?
2. Are there specific areas or skills you'd like to improve in your caregiving role, and how can you go about acquiring the necessary knowledge or training you need?

Closing Prayer:

Heavenly Father, when we find ourselves in unexpected caregiving roles, we sometimes doubt our abilities we ask You for wisdom in our time of need so that we can carry out our role in a most excellent way. Help us to remember that through Your strength, we can overcome any challenge. Guide us to seek training, lean on professionals, and prioritize self-care as we embrace these roles with open arms. As the North Star guided ancient travelers, guide us in our caregiving journey. In Jesus Name Amen.

Your Thoughts:

Day 16: Harmony in Balance

CARING FOR YOURSELF WHILE CARING FOR OTHERS

"You shall love your neighbor as yourself." - Mark 12:31 (ESV)

Hello hardy caregivers, and welcome to Day 16 of our journey. Today, we're addressing a delicate dance that many caregivers perform – finding balance between personal needs and caregiving responsibilities. In your multitasking world, don't forget the task of caring for your own needs.

Mark 12:31 reminds us to love our neighbor as ourselves. This includes the neighbor within you. Caring for yourself isn't selfish; it's an act of love and self-compassion.

Ralph Marston's words encourage us to rest when we're weary, to refresh and renew ourselves. It's like taking a deep breath before diving back into the waves. Self-care isn't a luxury; it's a necessity.

And always remember, caregivers, your well-being is like the sunshine that nurtures the garden of your heart. When you're nourished, you can continue to bloom and provide care with love and vitality.

I had to learn this the hard way. I didn't use wisdom and take the time to rest when I should have and needed to, so my ailing body got through to me instead. I did it to myself; drove myself twice over the last 25 years and had to be hospitalized due to exhaustion.

Sometimes, overdoing it takes its toll on us emotionally and, at times, physically. In my case, it was both. Believe me, I learned from the mistakes that led me there. I'm way more in touch with my body and soul than I was back in those days. I know when to pull back, quiet myself, and rest. Something I didn't do when I was younger. I don't drive myself like that anymore. Those times taught me to protect myself and set healthier boundaries. For me, it's always hard work to slow myself down. It's like putting the brakes on when sailing full speed down a hill. Nevertheless, if I want to live the way God wants me to live, I have to stop before I crash. I call it laboring to enter into God's rest.

Practical Applications:

1. Schedule "Me" Time: Dedicate regular slots in your schedule for self-care activities, whether it's reading, exercising, or pursuing a hobby.
2. Seek Support: Don't hesitate to ask for help from friends, family, or support groups to ensure you have time for yourself.
3. Release Guilt: Remind yourself that taking care of your well-being ultimately benefits your loved one. Release any guilt you may feel about prioritizing self-care.

Questions for Reflection:

1. How can you strike a harmonious balance between your personal needs and caregiving responsibilities without feeling guilty or inadequate?
2. What self-care activities bring you the most joy and rejuvenation, and how can you incorporate them into your routine?

Closing Prayer:

Heavenly Father, as caregivers striving to balance personal needs and caregiving responsibilities, we often wrestle with guilt and inadequacy. But we remember Your command to love ourselves as we love our neighbors. Grant us the wisdom to schedule "me" time, seek support, and release guilt, knowing that self-care is an act of love. In Jesus Name Amen.

Your Thoughts:

Day 17: Embracing Emotions

NAVIGATING THE HEART'S COMPLEX TERRAIN OF FEELINGS

"The LORD is near to the brokenhearted and saves the crushed in spirit." - Psalm 34:18 (ESV)

How are you today, Sensitive caregivers? Welcome to Day 17 of our incredible journey. Today, we're diving into the intricate world of emotions – the guilt, resentment, and other challenging feelings that can swell within us. It's like riding the waves of your heart, but remember, you're the fearless surfer.

Psalm 34:18 reminds us that the Lord is near to the brokenhearted. In moments of emotional turbulence, know that you're not alone. The One who created the oceans of your heart is with you.

Jonatan Mårtensson's analogy paints a vivid picture comparing feelings to waves. He points out that they come and go. Then he tells us that we have the power to choose which ones to surf and ride. It's a reminder that you can push through your emotions with wisdom from above and decide whether to be overtaken by the emotion or to overtake it like the fearless surfer does.

It is so important for us to embrace the transformative power of pure love and honesty in your caregiving journey. Release guilt and fear, allowing love to be your guiding light.

> "Feelings are much like waves; we can't stop them from coming, but we can choose which ones to surf."
> - Jonatan Mårtensson

Practical Applications:

Explore practical ways to shift your caregiving approach from guilt-driven to love-driven. Seek support, engage in self-care, and surround yourself with a loving community that can help you navigate the challenges of caregiving.

- Practice Emotional Awareness: Take time to identify and acknowledge your emotions. Understanding your feelings is the first step toward navigating the complex terrain of your heart.
- Develop Healthy Outlets: Find healthy ways to express and release your emotions. This could include journaling, talking to a trusted friend, or engaging in activities that bring you joy.

Questions for Reflection:

1. How do you currently approach and manage your emotions in your caregiving journey?
2. In what ways can you shift from fear-driven reactions to love-driven responses in your caregiving responsibilities?
3. How can you cultivate a healthy relationship with your own emotions and, in turn, model emotional well-being for those you care for?

. . .

Your Thoughts:

Day 18: Harmony in the Family

OVERCOMING CONFLICT WITH LOVE

"A new command I give you: Love one another. As I have loved you, so you must love one another." - John 13:34 (NIV)

Welcome, dedicated caregivers, to Day 18 of our remarkable journey. Today, we're tackling a common challenge that many caregivers face – handling conflicts with siblings and other family members while providing care for a loved one. When you're the primary caregiver your loved one has entrusted, it can sometimes feel like you're attempting to orchestrate a complex symphony with discordant notes. The differing opinions and sometimes off-key remarks from other relatives may lead you into the temptation of arguments. However, in these moments, it's crucial to wield the conductor's baton of love. Our goal is to harmonize these diverse notes, with the hope of creating a beautiful melody of care and support. Always remember, caregivers, in the symphony of your family, love is the conductor's baton that leads to a harmonious melody. Let it guide your interactions with grace and compassion.

John 13:34 reminds us of Jesus' command to love one another as He loved us. In times of conflict, let love guide your interactions. Love has the power to heal wounds and bridge divides.

Eva Burrows beautifully likens love to the oil that eases friction in family life. When conflict arises, remember that love is the bond that holds you together, like cement. It's the music that brings harmony back to your family's symphony.

> "In family life, love is the oil that eases friction,
> the cement that binds closer together,
> and the music that brings harmony."
> - Eva Burrows

Practical Applications:

1. Open Communication: Initiate calm and honest conversations with your siblings and family members. Share your perspectives and listen to theirs.
2. Set Boundaries: Establish clear boundaries and expectations regarding caregiving responsibilities to prevent misunderstandings.
3. Seek Mediation: If conflicts persist, consider involving a mediator, counselor, or family therapist to facilitate productive discussions.

Questions for Reflection:

1. How can you navigate conflicts with your siblings and family members in a way that reflects love and promotes harmony in your caregiving journey?
2. Are there specific communication strategies or boundaries you can implement to address conflicts more effectively?

Closing Prayer:

Heavenly Father, when conflicts arise with our siblings and family members in the midst of caregiving, we seek Your guidance. Help us remember Your command to love one another. Guide us to open communication, set healthy boundaries, and seek mediation when needed. May love be the oil, cement, and music that bring harmony to our family life. Amen.

Your Thoughts:

Day 19: Standing Strong

EMBRACING YOUR CAREGIVING CHOICES WITH
CONFIDENCE

"Why do you see the speck that is in your brother's eye, but
do not notice the log that is in your own eye?" - Matthew
7:3 (ESV)

Hello, steadfast caregivers, and welcome to Day 19 of
this sometimes-tumultuous journey. Today, we're
looking at another uncomfortable aspect of caregiving that we often face – feeling judged for our decisions and
the way we provide care. It's like walking through a field of
questions, but remember, we have the answers within us.

Matthew 7:3 reminds us of the tendency to notice specks in
others' eyes while overlooking logs in our own. When people
question your choices, remember that their perspective may
be clouded by their own experiences and beliefs. Just make
sure you're not the one with the log in your own eye trying to
remove the speck from theirs.

The anonymous quote offers a powerful reminder – people
will judge you regardless of your actions. So, forget the noise
and embrace your caregiving choices with confidence. You're

the one walking this path, and you know what's best for your loved one.

And always remember, caregivers, you are the best advocate for your loved one. Your decisions are made with love, and that's the most powerful guide of all.

> "People are going to judge you anyway,
> so forget everyone and be yourself."
> - Unknown

Practical Applications:

1. Self-Reflection: Take time for self-reflection to ensure your caregiving decisions align with your values and priorities.
2. Educate Others: Share information about your caregiving responsibilities and choices with those who question you. Education can dispel misconceptions.
3. Lean on Support: Seek support from fellow caregivers who understand your journey. They can offer empathy and advice on dealing with judgment.

Questions for Reflection:

1. How can you stand strong and embrace your caregiving choices with confidence, even when others question your priorities or motives?
2. Are there specific resources or support networks you can turn to when facing judgment for your caregiving decisions?

Closing Prayer:

Heavenly Father, when we feel judged for our caregiving decisions, it can be disheartening. But we remember the wisdom in Matthew 7:3 and the power of being true to ourselves. Help us reflect on our choices, educate others, and lean on the support of our caregiving community. Grant us the confidence to walk our path with grace and assurance. In Jesus Name Amen.

Affirmation:

"I embrace my caregiving choices with confidence, guided by love and the wisdom that comes from within. I am the best advocate for my loved one, and my decisions are made with purpose and compassion."

Your Thoughts:

Day 20: It's No Picnic

WHEN YOU FEEL LIKE CAVING IN

"I have told you these things so that in me you may have peace. In this world, you will have trouble. But take heart! I have overcome the world." - John 16:33

Taking care of an ornery, difficult loved one is no picnic. To say that an experience, task, person, or activity is no picnic means that it is quite difficult or unpleasant. I think back to a scene on the Andy Griffith Show when Andy, Barney, and their girlfriends left a nicely organized picnic to explore a cave. They were having fun until they got themselves into trouble. The walls caved in, and they found themselves trapped. It was no picnic. This can happen to caregivers who face tough issues with their loved ones. Since they are not experienced medical professionals, they may struggle to pull through and get out of the mess. BUT GOD will come through for them IF they trust, listen, and obey the way out of the mess. God knows the way out of the wilderness. All we have to do is follow. Caregivers can get stuck when things start falling down around them, just like when the walls of the cave collapse, blocking the way. When that happens, it is no picnic, as the saying goes. Andy, Barney, and the girls left the fun picnic and ended up in a not-so-fun predicament. God saved the day, just as God will save the day for us when we are in a tight spot.

"Challenges are what make life interesting,
and overcoming them is what makes life meaningful."
- Joshua J. Marine

Practical Applications:

1. Reflect on the challenges you've faced in caregiving. How have you felt stuck in difficult situations?
2. Trust that, like Andy and his friends, you can find a way out with God's guidance and support.
3. Consider how the promise from Romans 8:37 applies to your caregiving journey. You are more than a conqueror in Christ's love.

Questions for Reflection:

1. How has your caregiving journey felt like being trapped in a challenging situation?
2. In what ways has God provided a way out, similar to the rescue in the Andy Griffith episode?

Closing Prayer:

Dear Heavenly Father, we face difficulties in our caregiving journey that can feel like we're trapped in a collapsing cave. But we trust in your promise that we can overcome through Christ's love. Grant us the wisdom to listen, the strength to obey, and the faith to follow the way out. Just as you saved the day for Andy and his friends, we believe you will save the day for us in our times of need. In Jesus name, we pray, amen.

Affirmation:

I find strength in Christ's love to overcome caregiving challenges and with God's guidance, I will successfully navigate difficult situations that stand in my way.

Your Thoughts:

Day 21: Climb Through the Rubble

"Trust in the Lord with all your heart, and do not lean on your own understanding." - Proverbs 3:5

Today, I'm going to continue a little more on what I talked about yesterday. Believe me when I tell you, I know what it's like to care for cranky, angry, and difficult-to-deal-with loved ones. Some are deeply appreciative and kind, while others are ill-tempered, mean and unappreciative. Taking care of Mr. or Mrs. Crankenstein is far from a picnic. It can be extremely unpleasant, to say the least. However, these challenging moments are when we must look to God for wisdom and strength. Love will always come through if we keep believing and refuse to give up. Keep your chin and cheer up. Cheer yourself on. You can figure it out. Keep on keeping on until you get the victory.

When thinking about life not being a picnic, I again recall that scene from an old episode of "The Andy Griffith Show" when Andy, Barney, and the girls left behind a perfectly organized picnic to explore a mysterious old cave. They were having a great time exploring until the cave walls came crashing around them, leaving them trapped and gripped by fear. This situation was no picnic for them. Their only means of escape demanded they navigate through the intimidating rubble obstructing their path. The jumbled mess served as a daunting barrier, testing their resolve and determination.

Caregivers often come face to face with the prickly behaviors of irritable loved ones who are hard to deal with. When this happens, may we remember that in some way God will sustain us while we find the escape route. Our escape route might just appear as we quietly meditate on today's scripture verses or inspiring quotes. Maybe it will come from a song we recall in our heart or as we offer up the sacrifice of thanksgiving while it is going on around us. Either way, God will come through for us somehow if we listen for that still small voice and remain calm.

In these demanding moments, we turn to God for His divine intervention, akin to how He aided Andy of Mayberry and his friends in their need. Thankfully, they managed to extricate themselves from their predicament, and we can do the same. We will make it out even when life's circumstances close in around us, the walls of a cave collapse, and our way is blocked. It's essential to remember that, just as God was there for them in their hour of need, He stands ready to rescue us when we, too, find ourselves in a tight spot.

"Tough times never last, but tough people do."
- Robert H. Schuller

Practical Applications:

1. Reflect on a challenging caregiving situation you've faced. How did you find the wisdom and strength to overcome it?

2. In moments of doubt or difficulty, trust in the Lord with all your heart, seeking His guidance.

Questions for Reflection:

1. Can you share a time when you leaned on your faith to navigate a difficult caregiving challenge?
2. How can the experience of Andy, Barney, and their girlfriends in the cave relate to your caregiving journey?
3. How have faith and perseverance played a role in your own caregiving journey?
4. How were you able to overcome difficult moments with God's guidance?

Closing Prayer:

Heavenly Father, we come before you seeking wisdom and strength to navigate the challenging path of caregiving. Just as Andy, Barney, and their friends found a way out of their predicament, we trust in your guidance and support. In difficult moments, help us remember that love will always come through if we keep believing and refuse to give up. In Jesus name, we pray, amen.

Affirmations:

I can do all things through Christ who strengthens me, even in the face of caregiving challenges. I trust in the Lord with all my heart and find strength in Him when caregiving becomes challenging.

Your Thoughts:

Day 22: In Confusing Times

THE GOOD SHEPHERD BRINGS US BACK

"We all, like sheep, have gone astray, each of us has turned to our own way; and the Lord has laid on him the iniquity of us all." - Isaiah 53:6

L ife can sometimes take us down confusing and uncertain paths, much like a lost sheep that has strayed from the flock. In these moments, it's easy to feel overwhelmed, bewildered, and without a clear way forward. But, as followers of Christ, we have the assurance that God is our Shepherd. He is always happy to lead and guide us back to safety when we've gone astray. In today's devotional, we'll explore the promise that "God Makes a Way When There Seems to Be No Way."

Isaiah 53:6 reminds us that we, like sheep, often wander from God's intended path. We make mistakes, turn to our ways, and sometimes end up feeling lost and confused. Yet, this verse assures us that the Lord, in His boundless love, has taken upon Himself our iniquities.

When life's circumstances are confusing and off track, acknowledge that it's a common human experience just like we are told in 1 Corinthians 10:13. when facing trials, knowing that God is faithful and provides a way to endure and overcome.

Even when it seems impossible and bewildering we can ask for God's guidance and direction and He will lead us to a good place.

Practical Applications:

Seek Divine Wisdom: When faced with confusion and uncertainty, turn to God in prayer. Ask for wisdom and guidance, trusting that He generously provides direction without finding fault.

1. **Acknowledge Common Experiences:**
   Understand that facing confusing and off-track situations is a common human experience, as mentioned in 1 Corinthians 10:13. Recognize that you are not alone in your struggles, and God is faithful to provide a way to endure and overcome.
2. **Ask for Guidance:** Just as a lost sheep would depend on its shepherd for direction, ask God for His guidance and direction when you feel lost and bewildered. Trust that He will lead you to a good place, even when the path seems unclear.

Questions for Reflection:

1. In what ways have you experienced moments when life seemed confusing and off track?
2. How can you apply the promise from Isaiah 53:6, James 1:5, and 1 Corinthians 10:13 to your current circumstances?

Closing Prayer:

Dear Heavenly Father, in the midst of life's confusing and uncertain moments, we turn to You as our Shepherd. We trust that even when we've strayed, You will make a way when there seems to be no way. We seek Your wisdom and guidance, knowing that You generously provide direction without finding fault. Thank you for your love, care, and the promise of finding the way when we're lost. We also thank you for the promise that you will provide a way to endure and overcome trials. In Jesus' name, we pray, amen.

Affirmation:

I will trust when the path is unclear and I will rely on God's wisdom to steer me through frightening situations.

Your Thoughts:

Day 23: Safety First

PROTECTING OUR LOVED ONES FROM THEMSELVES

"For he will command his angels concerning you to guard you in all your ways." - Psalm 91:11

Hail, Valiant Caregivers! You stalwart protectors of our dear ones who can no longer shield themselves. We are the Safety Patrol and we must approach this task with love and a dash of empathy. Through proactive measures and open chats, we keep our loved ones snug. Yet, some elders dodge guidance, turning our caregiving journey into a labor-intensive comedy sketch. We caregivers end up adopting a hawk-eyed stance, making sure safety rules aren't treated like optional snacks. Nope, our loved ones must eat the whole meal we're serving them. We work at balancing autonomy and safety. We intervene with a gentle but firm nudge. As guardians, we must insist on safety without dulling their sparkle, all fueled by care and love. Communication, our superhero tool, involves expressing concern with a sprinkle of humor. It's always about finding a way to balance respect for their autonomy while ensuring safety. All this means we have to watch our beloved like a vigilant hawk. Believe me when I say that this is something I have to deal with every day and it gets tiring. As much as I like hawks, it's hard trying to be one myself.

"Protecting someone's welfare isn't about restricting their freedom; it's about preserving their safety and well-being."
- Unknown

Practical Applications:

1. Engage in open and honest conversations with your loved one about safety concerns. Discuss the reasons behind certain safety measures and decisions.
2. Take proactive steps to reduce potential hazards.
3. Seek guidance from healthcare professionals, counselors, or support groups if your loved one's safety is a consistent concern. They can provide valuable insights and strategies.

Questions for Reflection:

1. How do you balance respecting your loved one's autonomy while ensuring their safety?
2. In what ways can you communicate your care and protection to your loved one, so they understand your intentions are out of love and not control?

Closing Prayer:

Heavenly Father, we come before you with hearts filled with love and concern for our dear ones. We want to protect their welfare and safety. Grant us the wisdom to have open conversations and implement practical measures to ensure their well-being. May we strike a balance between allowing them independence and providing protection. In Jesus' name, we pray. Amen.

Your Thoughts:

Day 24: Creative Caregiving

HANDLING THOSE TRICKY SITUATIONS

"If any of you lacks wisdom, you should ask God, who gives generously to all without finding fault, and it will be given to you." - James 1:5

Hello Creative Caregivers. Today is Day 24 and it's the day to address Tricky Situations that arise. As a family caregiver, you may face moments where traditional communication and reasoning are insufficient. This is especially true when your loved one is cognitively impaired. Occasionally, there are situations where guiding or persuading your elderly loved one proves ineffective, jeopardizing their safety. In such moments like these, you may want to consider two valuable strategies as a last resort. Using "therapeutic lying" or "playing make-believe," as I call it might be the answer when you're in this kind of pickle. This method can involve providing information that's not entirely accurate to protect your loved one when their judgment is impaired, ensuring their safety and well-being. While it should be used with caution and as a last resort, it can be a compassionate approach to maintain their independence and protect them from harm.

I believe that there are instances when this strategy works like a miracle cure fix for a distressing situation. When there is no other way to reason, this strategy works wonders to redirect your loved one away from what otherwise would make them become more distraught. It's definitely a de-escalator. You may also use this method to prevent them from physical harm. With an already confused individual, I see no reason to upset the apple cart any more than it is already upset. You might even amaze yourself with the stories you conjure up when you let your own creative juices flow.

At this time I want to share a certain technique that usually works when nothing else does. Now, here's the technique I've found to be incredibly helpful in my caregiving journey. I like to call it the "Imagination Technique."

Picture this: you're with your loved one, and they have a unique perspective on things. But you know their reality might not align with the facts. That's when you put on your creative hat and dive headfirst into their world of wonderful imagination. It's like a grand adventure into a world of make-believe!

And here's the fun part: you're not lying; you're crafting stories, much like a pro storyteller. You're turning confusion into clarity and anxiety into smiles. It's as if you're a master problem solver, ensuring your loved one stays safe and happy.

But, my friend, remember, it's not just about caregiving; it's about crafting moments of joy and understanding. It's a technique that turns those off-kilter days into moments of caregiving wonder.

You see, I've been there, done that, and trust me, it works wonders. It's a secret weapon for caregivers who turn challenges into opportunities for laughter and love. Laughter and imagination make the best combo!

So, when things get a bit unique in your caregiving world, just remember the "Imagination Technique." It's your personal touch of caregiving brilliance!

Some professionals call this strategy "Therapeutic Lying": I liken it to the compassionate choices made by Rahab and the Hebrew midwives. Just as they acted to protect lives and fulfill a higher purpose, caregivers may use therapeutic lying to prevent distress or harm to their loved ones. This approach prioritizes safety and well-being while honoring the reality perceived by individuals with cognitive impairments. It's a last-resort option, used with caution, to maintain a loved one's safety, well-being, and dignity.

I prefer to call it Playing Make-Believe: As a child I absolutely loved playing make believe. It's a great way of entering into the world as perceived by the person who has a cognitive impairment. Caregivers entering into the world of imagination can create a safe and supportive environment without arguments. All you have to be is good at making up a good story. It is simply a form of role-playing. Instead of seeing it as being dishonest, realize that you are helping to create a comforting and secure environment, promoting emotional well-being, and helping navigate the challenges of cognitive decline. I assure you, it works wonders for dispelling frustration.

Think of these strategies as the VIP treatment for your loved ones' emotions. It's like rolling out the red carpet for their well-being, complete with safety, independence, and a sprinkle of joy.

"You have two hands, one to help yourself,
the second to help others."
- Audrey Hepburn

Practical Applications:

1. **Approach with Empathy:** Embrace "therapeutic lying" and/or "playing make-believe" as tools to support your loved one's emotional well-being and keep them safe.
2. **Use with Caution:** Apply these strategies as a last resort, always prioritizing honesty and open communication when possible.
3. **Seek Guidance:** If you are uncomfortable with this technique consult with healthcare professionals or experts in gerontology to evaluate the appropriateness of these approaches in specific situations.

Questions for Reflection:

1. How does viewing "therapeutic lying" as a form of compassion and "playing make-believe" affect your perspective on caregiving strategies?
2. In what situations do you believe these approaches could be most beneficial for your loved one's well-being?
3. How do you feel about employing this modality in caregiving? What reservations or concerns do you have?
4. What circumstances would you consider appropriate for you to utilize this?

Closing Prayer:

Heavenly Father, guide us in making difficult decisions that prioritize the well-being of our loved ones. Help us navigate the challenges of caregiving with love, compassion, and integrity. May therapeutic lying and "playing make-believe" be tools of empathy and support in fostering safety, independence, and emotional well-being. In Jesus' name, we pray. Amen.

Affirmations:

"I approach caregiving with love and compassion, always seeking the best for my loved one. I prioritize the emotional well-being and safety of my loved one in all caregiving decisions. I seek guidance and support when facing challenging situations."

Your Thoughts:

Day 25: Tender Touch

NURTURING THE SOUL THROUGH PHYSICAL CONNECTION

"And Jesus, moved with compassion, touched their eyes, and immediately they regained their sight and followed Him." - Matthew 20:34

H ello, Caregiver Companions, and welcome to a day dedicated to the profound impact of touch in our caregiving journey. Today, we're exploring the gentle art of using touch as a powerful language of love and comfort.

In my own caregiving experience, I've witnessed the transformative power of touch. Whether it's a reassuring hand on the shoulder during a challenging moment or a gentle embrace to express love, touch has a unique way of communicating beyond words.

"Too often we underestimate the power of a touch,
a smile, a kind word, a listening ear, an honest compliment, or
the smallest act of caring, all of which have the potential to
turn a life around."
- Leo Buscaglia

"Your own hands can become the warm,
soothing hands of the Savior when you cherish,
love, and serve with pure intent."
- Dieter F. Uchtdorf

Practical Applications:

1. **The Healing Touch:** When appropriate, use touch to convey comfort. A hand on the shoulder or a gentle pat can speak volumes.
2. **Massage Moments:** Explore simple hand or foot massages as a way to provide physical comfort and relaxation.
3. **Hug it Out:** Embrace the power of a warm hug. Physical touch releases oxytocin, the "love hormone," promoting a sense of bonding and well-being.

Questions for Reflection:

1. How do you currently incorporate touch into your caregiving routine?
2. How do you feel about incorporating touch into your caregiving routine? Share your thoughts and experiences
3. Are there cultural or personal considerations that influence your approach to touch?
4. In what ways can you be more intentional about using touch as a means of communication and comfort?

Closing Prayer:

Heavenly Father, we thank you for the gift of touch, a language of love that transcends words. As caregivers, may our hands be instruments of comfort, our embraces be a source of solace, and our touch reflect the warmth of your love. In Jesus' name, we pray. Amen.

Affirmation:

"I will use the language of touch to communicate love, comfort, and compassion in my caregiving journey."

Your Thoughts:

Day 26: Keeping the JOY in the Journey

MIRTH-FILLED MOMENTS

"A cheerful heart is good medicine, but a crushed spirit dries up the bones." - Proverbs 17:22

Hello Chuckling Caregivers. Welcome to Day 26 of our transformative journey. Today is the day we're exploring the remarkable influence of laughter and joy in our caregiving roles. It's like finding a treasure chest in the midst of life's challenges, and you hold the key.

In the whirlwind of caregiving, we often discover that humor can be a balm for the soul, a source of strength that lightens our hearts amid the challenges. This day is dedicated to the joy that laughter brings and the profound impact it has on both the caregiver and the one receiving care.

One thing I am is nutty. Even one of the meanings of my name Evelyn means hazelnut. I love instilling humor into my care. As a nurse, one of my hallmark qualities has been recognizing that a well-timed laugh can be a total blessing to my patients, especially when they're dealing with serious health situations.

While there are countless reasons to enjoy a good laugh. I have a never-ending list of funny stories to tell, but I won't delve into them now. Just know that laughter is a vital tool for healing. The things I have done and do just to get a laugh are do make a world of difference in an otherwise boring day.

Do your best to enter into the world of levity and humor and you will experience the best caregiving and life has to offer.

"Laughter is an instant vacation."
- Milton Berle

Practical Application:

1. **Comedic Relief Routine:** Introduce a daily dose of humor, whether it's through a funny story, a light-hearted movie, or a good joke. Laughter can be a powerful stress-reliever. Create a routine that includes moments of lightness to break up the day. You might think of investing your money into book of jokes. Sometimes I read jokes to my loved one and it brings out the best in them.

2. **Create a Laughter Journal:** Document moments of joy and humor during your caregiving journey. Reflecting on these moments can be a source of encouragement during tougher times. Share this journal with others, spreading the joy.

3. **Share Laughter with Your Loved One:** Find activities or shows that bring joy to both you and your loved one. Whether it's a favorite comedy show or reminiscing about funny memories, shared laughter can strengthen your bond and create positive moments.

Questions for Reflection:

1. How do you currently incorporate humor into your caregiving routine, and how has it impacted your overall well-being?
2. In what ways can you bring more laughter into your caregiving environment, both for yourself and your loved one?
3. Reflect on a specific moment when laughter transformed a challenging situation. How can you recreate such moments intentionally?
4. Think about moments of joy you have discovered. How has laughter brought joy to your caregiving days?

Closing Prayer:

Dear Heavenly Father, in the midst of our caregiving journey, we acknowledge the gift of laughter, a medicine for the soul. Grant us the wisdom to find joy in the midst of challenges, to share laughter with our loved ones, and to cultivate a spirit of humor that lightens the load. May our homes be filled with the sounds of laughter and joy. In Jesus' name, we pray. Amen.

Affirmation:

"I embrace the gift of laughter in my caregiving journey. Through joy and humor, I find strength, resilience, and a deeper connection with my loved one."

Your Thoughts:

Day 27: The Disorderly Digestion Dilemma

WHEN THE GOING GETS TOUGH

"The Lord sustains them on their sickbed and restores them from their bed of illness." - Psalm 41:3

Hello, Responsive Caregivers, and welcome to Day 27. Today, we're addressing a topic that often presents itself in the caregiving realm – constipation. It's an aspect of disorderly digestion that requires careful consideration and compassionate actions. As caregivers, understanding and managing constipation are vital components of providing holistic care to our loved ones. The number of times I've stepped in to assist individuals grappling with this challenging condition is known only to the Lord. While there are numerous stories I could share about such situations, those tales will have to wait for another time. It's enough to say that, as a nurse, I've been repeatedly called upon over the years to offer compassionate assistance to those struggling to relieve themselves. In fact, I'm so at it that I've affectionately earned the nickname 'Fannie Freedom' for my proficiency in aiding individuals in overcoming this turtle hurdle.

"Patience is not the ability to wait,
but the ability to keep a good attitude while waiting."
- Joyce Meyer

Practical Applications:

Dietary Considerations: Collaborate with healthcare professionals to design a diet that promotes regular bowel movements. Each person is so individualized. What works for one might not work for another.

1. Be diligent in monitoring your loved one's bowel movements.Establishing Routine.
2. It's best not to let your loved one stall more than 3 days.
3. Create a consistent daily routine that includes time for toileting. Predictable routines can help regulate bowel movements.
4. Consult your healthcare provider if constipation persists, seek guidance their guidance. They can recommend appropriate medications, supplements or other interventions to alleviate the issue.

Questions for Reflection:

1. How can you adjust your loved one's diet to include more fiber and promote digestive health?
2. In what ways can you establish a daily routine that supports regular toileting for your loved one?
3. Have you consulted with healthcare professionals to address persistent constipation issues?

Closing Prayer:

Heavenly Father, as we navigate the challenges of constipation, we turn to You for guidance and strength. Grant us the wisdom to make dietary adjustments, establish supportive routines, and seek medical advice when needed. May Your comforting presence sustain us in these caregiving moments. In Jesus' name, we pray. In Jesus Name Amen.

Affirmation:

"I approach constipation challenges with compassion and diligence, seeking solutions with the guidance of healthcare professionals and the sustaining grace of the Lord."

Your Thoughts:

Day 28: In the Embrace of Grace

LOVE, FAITH, AND LOGIC IN END-OF-LIFE DECISIONS

"For I know the plans I have for you, declares the LORD, plans for welfare and not for evil, to give you a future and a hope." - Jeremiah 29:11 (ESV)

W elcome to Day 28, Compassionate Caregiver. Today we will go into making end-of-life decisions. This is where the intersection of faith, logic and caregiving meet. It's smart and wise to prepare and talk about this subject even though it's one of the more difficult subjects to discuss. It should, however, be done. Preparing for your loved one's celestial discharge from this earth will occur. We can rest assured that the inevitable will occur. It's easy to be swayed by emotions when making decisions for our loved ones, but combining faith in God's plan with logical thinking can lead to the best outcomes. Jeremiah 29:11 reminds us that the Lord has plans for our welfare and a future filled with hope. In the challenging realm of end-of-life decisions, trust that there is guidance and purpose in every choice you make. Seneca's words also encourage us not to be deterred by the difficulty of decisions but to dare to face them. The path to making end-of-life decisions is filled with uncertainties, but your love and courage will light the way. Look unto Jesus who is THE Light and the author and finisher of our faith. He will show you the way because He is also The Way.

The Following are Some Examples of Faith and Logic:

Treatment Choice: A caregiver was faced with deciding on the appropriate treatment for their loved one's chronic illness. They carefully researched various treatment options, considering success rates, potential side effects, and expert opinions. While they emotionally desired a quick fix, their logical approach led them to a treatment that was more effective in the long run, ultimately improving their loved one's health.

Care Transition: When the time came for their loved one to transition to a care facility, a caregiver faced mixed emotions. Although they were emotionally attached to the idea of providing care at home, they logically assessed their loved one's needs and the professional care required. They made the difficult but logical decision to move their loved one to a care facility where they received the specialized care needed for their condition. This choice resulted in a safer and more comfortable environment.

End-of-Life Care: In the final stages of their loved one's life, a caregiver had to make decisions about palliative care and end-of-life choices. Emotions were high, but they combined faith in God's plan with logical decision-making. They created an advanced care plan, ensuring that their loved one's wishes were respected, which brought peace to their loved one's final days and prevented unnecessary emotional burdens.

. . .

Some Encouraging Words for You Today:

Remember that your caregiving journey is guided by faith in God's ultimate plan and logical decision-making. This powerful combination can lead to better care, both physically and emotionally.

"The intersection of faith and logic is where miracles happen in caregiving. When you trust and think, you can make the best decisions for your loved one."
- Unknown

Practical Applications:

1. Conversations: Have open and honest conversations with your loved one about their wishes and values regarding end-of-life care.
2. Medical Information: Seek information from healthcare professionals to understand your loved one's medical condition, treatment options, and prognosis.
3. Advance Directives: Familiarize yourself with advance directives like living wills and durable power of attorney for healthcare. These legal documents can provide clarity on your loved one's preferences.

Questions for Reflection:

1. How can you approach end-of-life decisions with love, compassion, and a commitment to honoring your loved one's wishes?
2. Are there resources or professionals who can assist you in making informed end-of-life decisions?

Closing Prayer:

Heavenly Father, as we begin the discussion on end-of-life decisions, we seek Your guidance and wisdom. Help us trust in Your plans for welfare and hope. Grant us the courage to have meaningful conversations, seek medical information, and explore advance directives. May love always be our guiding light in these profound moments.

We thank you for the wisdom to combine faith and logic in our caregiving roles. Guide us in making choices that align with your plan and bring comfort and healing to our loved ones. We trust you as we walk this path of faith and logic. In Jesus Name Amen.

Affirmation:

"Today, I affirm my commitment to approach end-of-life decisions with a heart full of love, unwavering faith, and clear-headed wisdom. I trust that guided by these principles, I can navigate this sacred journey with grace and compassion."

Your Thoughts:

Day 29: Sunshine Chats

BRIGHTENING YOUR LOVED ONE'S DAY WITH CONVERSATION

"Pleasant words are a honeycomb, sweet to the soul and healing to the bones." - Proverbs 16:24

I t's a great day, Compassionate Caregivers! We're one day away from the end of our 30-day journey, and it's time to focus on the art of positive and uplifting conversations with our elderly loved ones. As caregivers, our role extends beyond physical care; we're also stewards of their emotional well-being.

In a world often filled with distressing global events, our elderly loved ones may feel a sense of powerlessness. Today's devotion focuses on maintaining light and positive conversations, providing a safe haven from the weight of the world.

Through countless heart-to-heart talks with my elderly loved ones, I've discovered a treasure trove of joyous memories. It's truly enchanting when these conversations become the catalyst for laughter, infusing a burst of vibrancy into what might otherwise be a mundane day. Even when they revisit the challenges of the Great Depression or the tumultuous World War era, the very act of sharing those experiences fills them with a sense of accomplishment. Most importantly, they appreciate being heard; it's a two-way street where every shared story weaves a unique tapestry of life.

In the art of dialogue, it's clear that our elders not only have stories to tell but a profound desire to share them. This exchange isn't just a recounting of the past; it's a living, breathing narrative that transcends time. It's a dance of shared moments, offering insights into a life richly lived.

Contrary to misguided beliefs, the elderly aren't silent observers of history; they are animated storytellers, each tale a brushstroke contributing to the masterpiece of their experiences. Every shared moment reinforces why they are still a vital part of our lives and why their stories continue to shape the world. In essence, our elders are not merely keepers of memories; they are architects of a legacy that adds depth and meaning to the fabric of our shared existence.

"The simple act of caring is heroic."
- Edward Albert

Practical Application:

1. Discover Their Interests: Engage your loved one in discussions about their personal experiences, hobbies, or favorite pastimes. Discovering what brings them joy can lead to meaningful conversations.
2. Share Light-Hearted Current Events: Instead of delving into heavy topics, discuss uplifting current events related to entertainment, nature, or positive community stories. This fosters a sense of connection and joy.
3. Reflect on Fond Memories: Encourage your loved one to share fond memories from their past.

Reflecting on positive experiences not only brings joy but also stimulates cognitive functioning.

Questions for Reflection:

1. What topics or activities bring the most joy and engagement to your loved one?
2. How can you incorporate more positive conversations into your daily interactions?
3. What memories or experiences can you revisit with your loved one to evoke feelings of joy and fulfillment?

Closing Prayer:

Heavenly Father, guide our conversations with our elderly loved ones. Grant us the wisdom to focus on positive and uplifting topics that bring joy and comfort. May our interactions be a source of light and happiness, nurturing their emotional well-being. In Jesus' name, we pray Amen.

Affirmation:

"I choose to fill our conversations with joy and positivity, creating a nurturing space for my loved one's emotional well-being."

Your Thoughts:

Day 30: When the Day Comes

HONORING MEMORIES

"Blessed are those who mourn, for they shall be comforted." - Matthew 5:4 (ESV)

Hello, servant-hearted caregivers, and welcome to Day 30. Today, we delve into a profound and universal experience – grief and loss. It's like walking through a valley of memories, but remember, love is the lantern that lights your way.

Matthew 5:4 reminds us that those who mourn shall be comforted. In moments of grief, know that comfort and solace are not distant. They are present, embracing you like a warm hug.

Queen Elizabeth II beautifully acknowledges that grief is the price we pay for love. The depth of our sorrow reflects the depth of our love. It's a testament to the precious moments and connections we shared.

> "Grief is the price we pay for love."
> - Queen Elizabeth II

Practical Applications:

1. Allow Yourself to Grieve: Give yourself permission to grieve in your unique way. There's no right or wrong way to mourn.
2. Lean on Support: Seek support from friends, family, or grief support groups. Sharing your feelings can be profoundly healing.
3. Memorialize: Find meaningful ways to honor your loved one's memory, such as creating a memorial or participating in acts of kindness in their name.

Questions for Reflection:

1. How can you navigate the complex journey of grief and loss with love and self-compassion?
2. Are there specific rituals or ways you'd like to honor your loved one's memory and find comfort in the grieving process?

Closing Prayer:

Heavenly Father, as we conclude our journey, we turn to You for strength in times of grief and loss. Bless those who mourn, and may they find comfort in Your embrace. Help us allow ourselves to grieve, lean on support, and find meaningful ways to honor our loved ones. May love always be our guiding light through the valley of memories. In Jesus Name Amen.

Affirmation:

"I embrace the memories of my loved ones, cherishing the moments we shared and finding strength in the legacy they've left behind. Today, I honor their lives with gratitude and love."

Your Thoughts:

About the Author

Evelyn's passion for nursing and the joy of selfless service ignited at the age of 13 during her early experiences as a volunteer 'Pinky' at the local hospital. Despite facing mockery and ridicule from some peers for working without pay, her commitment to comfort, care for, and serve others remained unwavering.

Over the years, along with her accolades and numerous civic honors, she has been the recipient of several prestigious awards, including The National Nurse Hero Award at the American Red Cross Headquarters in Washington, DC. She was concurrently featured on the cover of Nursing Spectrum Magazine, along with an article exemplifying her determination to preserve and protect lives. Additionally, she was granted The Making a Difference Award from the Russ Berrie Institute, an honor bestowed on unsung heroes living in New Jersey, specifically those whose outstanding community service and heroic acts have made a substantial impact on the lives of others. In his book *Selling From The Inside Out*, author Barry Siskind uses her as an example of someone who presses on in dire circumstances, using courage and hope to overcome perilous obstacles

Now a seasoned professional with 50 years of experience, she is a Certified Care Manager, Patient Advocate, Author, Educator, Speaker, and Humorist. Her true joy lies in the field of Aging Family Care, where she employs an Integrative Holistic

Nursing approach. Evelyn believes Christian believers have been created for good works in Christ. This is the reason why she offers herself to God daily, viewing what she does as an act of spiritual worship.

She is known for her proactive, tenacious approach to overcoming obstacles and her passion for sharing her 'Nurse-Wit.' Her vast clinical experience extends to caring not only for clients but also for their families. She was the primary caregiver for her own father, mother, and mother-in-law, and now an elderly aunt facing cognitive impairments.

Her mission is to enhance and maintain the quality of life for all and not just the elderly. She offers empathy and compassion to both seniors and families alike, navigating them through today's complicated healthcare system. Be assured that she deeply understands the pressures and joys of the 'Sandwich Generation.' She strives to help seniors stay safe and independent in the familiar surroundings of home where they prefer to live out their years. If, for some reason, a loved one must move into a facility, her job is to make their transition as smooth and seamless as possible while assisting their families in making those difficult decisions.

In addition to her nursing career, Evelyn pursued Massage Therapy, receiving her N.Y. State License. She served as Interim President of the National Association of Nurse Massage Therapists board and strongly advocates for the power of caring touch in patient care.

Ever the optimist, Evelyn has a Can-Do Attitude. Her lighthearted, amusing approach has earned her the name "Nurse Sunshine." She is available for speaking engagements and presents on many topics in Community and Professional settings.

She can be contacted at nursesunshine777@gmail.com.